Shalom Hirschman

The Changing Face of American Medicine

AF153262

Shalom Hirschman

The Changing Face of American Medicine

LAP LAMBERT Academic Publishing

Impressum / Imprint

Bibliografische Information der Deutschen Nationalbibliothek: Die Deutsche Nationalbibliothek verzeichnet diese Publikation in der Deutschen Nationalbibliografie; detaillierte bibliografische Daten sind im Internet über http://dnb.d-nb.de abrufbar.
Alle in diesem Buch genannten Marken und Produktnamen unterliegen warenzeichen-, marken- oder patentrechtlichem Schutz bzw. sind Warenzeichen oder eingetragene Warenzeichen der jeweiligen Inhaber. Die Wiedergabe von Marken, Produktnamen, Gebrauchsnamen, Handelsnamen, Warenbezeichnungen u.s.w. in diesem Werk berechtigt auch ohne besondere Kennzeichnung nicht zu der Annahme, dass solche Namen im Sinne der Warenzeichen- und Markenschutzgesetzgebung als frei zu betrachten wären und daher von jedermann benutzt werden dürften.

Bibliographic information published by the Deutsche Nationalbibliothek: The Deutsche Nationalbibliothek lists this publication in the Deutsche Nationalbibliografie; detailed bibliographic data are available in the Internet at http://dnb.d-nb.de.
Any brand names and product names mentioned in this book are subject to trademark, brand or patent protection and are trademarks or registered trademarks of their respective holders. The use of brand names, product names, common names, trade names, product descriptions etc. even without a particular marking in this works is in no way to be construed to mean that such names may be regarded as unrestricted in respect of trademark and brand protection legislation and could thus be used by anyone.

Coverbild / Cover image: www.ingimage.com

Verlag / Publisher:
LAP LAMBERT Academic Publishing
ist ein Imprint der / is a trademark of
OmniScriptum GmbH & Co. KG
Heinrich-Böcking-Str. 6-8, 66121 Saarbrücken, Deutschland / Germany
Email: info@lap-publishing.com

Herstellung: siehe letzte Seite /
Printed at: see last page
ISBN: 978-3-659-60784-4

The Changing Face of American Medicine

Shalom Z Hirschman, M.D.

Contents

Dedication and Prologue

I have written this book to honor my best friend of more than four decades, the late extraordinary educator Dr. Bernard Lander. The accomplishment of Dr. Lander's dream to establish a new school of higher education, an effort that he began in 1970, culminated in the purchase of the New York Medical College in 2010 just prior to his demise at age 94. I was his junior by 20 years but he pulled me with him on an exciting adventure in the creation of a college and institution of higher learning.

But why was the high point of this journey the purchase of a medical school? What is the special quality of a medical school that endows it with the power to become the ultimate quest of an innovative educator?

As I tell this tale of the vicissitudes of medical education and practice, the uniqueness of medicine and medical education as very humane and altruistic pursuits will become apparent. The fundamental objective of medicine is to serve other human beings both individually and collectively. Dr. Lander viewed education as a humane service, as an instrument for the betterment of each individual and for the provision of society as a whole at every level, with medical education representing the ultimate human endeavor.

In this volume I record my own views on the practice of medicine, biomedical research and teaching of both medical students and biomedical graduate students, honed by more than half a century in medical practice, teaching and research. Much of what I write had its origins in repeated discussions with colleagues, students, patients and with Dr. Lander as I helped to realize his many dreams in education.

The past 50 years have been a time of ferment in biomedical research. From the characterization of deoxyribonucleic acids as the mediators of genetic information, based on the tri-nucleotide code for each amino acid placed into a protein's peptide strand, a new informational revolution gathered strength and produced more knowledge about the biological world than had been gathered in previous millennia. Medicine is faced with the task of turning this information into practical usages for the treatment of disease and the preventive maintenance of human health.

Medical educators now must devise methods of breaking down this geometric progression of new basic biomedical knowledge into rudiments transmitted to students that would allow them to self – educate for the rest of their lives. The deciphering of the genetic code and the more recent advances in the technology of DNA sequencing have given birth to a new era of personalized genomic based medicine. Although this field is currently still in its early infancy one can expect that physicians increasingly will be bombarded with new data requiring new approaches to diagnosis and therapy. The packaging of this data so that it is useful and manageable by physicians will become an important educational task in the ensuing decades.

The quest for advances in medical knowledge must be continuously supported financially whether by government, private sector or philanthropic funding. The overhaul of medical practice and, pari passu, medical education by the Affordable Care Act passed by Congress in 2010 will result in new academic and financial challenges for medical schools, practicing physicians and biomedical researchers. As I recount my fifty year journey in an ever changing healthcare landscape, the reader will realize that I am confident that these challenges will be met in creative ways that will accrue to the benefit of mankind.

Chapter 1. Medicine During My Early Years

I first embarked on my journey through the landscape of medicine during my years of internship and residency in internal medicine, in the early 1960's, at The Massachusetts General Hospital, the world-renown teaching hospital of The Harvard Medical School. The code-words for medical practice as imbued by my mentors were dedication, hard work, perseverance, and absolute responsibility in the care of patients. The patient came first and was the focal point of the physician's life. Interns and residents (house officers) were on duty every other night and every other weekend but really worked day and night. Even on nights off one did not leave the hospital ward until open matters for every patient under care were addressed. House officers performed blood counts and microscopic examinations and urine examinations. Great pride was taken in learning how to perform procedures such as thoracentesis, pleural biopsy and bone marrow aspiration. Clinical teaching emphasized "hands-on" medicine.

Every patient entering the hospital emergency room was given thoughtful medical care without regard to social or ethnic status. The objective of clinical teaching was to ingrain the altruistic responsibilities of medical practice by the physician. The practice of medicine was in no way a 9-5 job; rather it was demanding, engrossing and all consuming. Spare moments were spent reading the medical literature and cogitating about medical problems presented by patients. Patient finances, insurance payments and cost of care were not matters that appeared during medical care conferences. A life dedicated to the practice of medicine required never ending self-education to stay abreast of advancing medical knowledge. Colleagues in the practice of medicine were expected to exhibit absolute dedication to care of patients and a continuous quest for increased knowledge of their field of medicine.

It is not my intent to idealize, or idolize, the era of my younger years in medicine. However, there is no doubt that the three decades spanning the 1950's through the

1970's witnessed the rise of American medicine to world supremacy in medical practice, medical teaching and medical research. The United States became the paragon and model country for proper care of patients, medical education and biomedical research. Much of the surge of the United States in medicine, especially in both basic and clinical medical research, was fueled by the federal government through liberal funding of the National Institutes of Health and the National Science Foundation who, in turn, funded biomedical research on a national scale.

Now I turn to considerations of present realities and my vision of the future of American medicine.

Chapter 2. My Academic Practice of Medicine in New York City

In early 1968, while I was engaged in basic research at the National Institutes of Health (NIH) in Bethesda, Maryland, my former schoolmate, Dr. Jesse Roth, who later became director of the diabetes section of the National Institutes of Arthritis and Metabolism, introduced me to Dr. Solomon Berson who had just been appointed as Chairman of the Department of Medicine at the new Mount Sinai School of Medicine in New York City. With his coworker, Dr. Rosalind Yalow, Dr. Berson had developed the radioimmunoassay to quantitatively measure peptides and proteins thereby opening up the field of peptide hormone biochemistry and endocrinology. Dr. Berson did not live to receive the Nobel laureate that was awarded for this work and was accepted by Dr. Yalow. (Several years later Dr.Yalow told me that her father was an orthodox rabbi and that she maintained a strictly kosher home. Dr. Yalow was admired for her culinary talents.) I was both awed and fascinated by Dr. Berson. He had a keen super quick mind that penetrated to the essence of a problem almost instantly. Dr. Berson came to the NIH in Bethesda to interview me. I met him in the Clinical Center building of the NIH and we walked the hall on the floor were Jesse Roth had his laboratory looking for an empty room. Dr. Berson opened a door. The room was empty but there were no chairs. He sat down on the floor and I followed suit. For almost three hours we talked about medicine, research, teaching, and his visions for the department of medicine at the world famous Mount Sinai Hospital that developed the new medical school. At the end of the session he offered me the position as director of the division of infectious diseases, with an appointment as associate professor in the medical school, and said that he wanted me to accept the offer right then and there. I just could not say no or even think it over. This is how I was appointed to become the youngest colleague of the leaders of a department of medicine that probably had the greatest assemblage of icons in the history of American medicine in a single department of medicine. My new colleagues, who were directors of the divisions of the department of medicine at The Mount Sinai Medical Center, had been my teachers either through their lectures when I was a student at the Albert Einstein College of Medicine or through the textbooks that they had authored and which I had read word for word during my student years in medical school and during my internship and residency years at the Massachusetts General Hospital.

I cannot forget the first division chiefs meeting of the department of medicine that I attended a few days after I moved to New York City in May of 1969. Sitting at the table were some of the most respected physicians not only in the United States but in the entire world. To my right was Dr. Charles Friedberg the world-renowned cardiologist whose comprehensive textbook on cardiology was the "only book to read" on the subject. Dr. Friedberg had agreed to step down as director of the division of cardiology and Dr. Berson had appointed Dr. Arnold Katz as the new director. Dr. Katz had not yet arrived in New York City so Dr. Friedberg was still serving as director. Dr. Katz was just a few years ahead of me in the internship and residency in internal medicine at the Massachusetts General Hospital and he was the son of a famous cardiologist who was an expert on the treatment of cardiac arrhythmias. Later on Dr. Katz would make the important discovery of calcium channels in the heart that led to the development of channel blocker drugs for the treatment of heart disease. Next to Dr. Friedberg sat Dr. Louis Siltzbach, the director of the division of pulmonary medicine, whose antigen preparation (Siltzbach-Kveim test) was used all over the world to help make the diagnosis of sarcoidosis. These elder statesmen of American medicine shaped the early years of the new Mount Sinai School of Medicine and were models of the previous generation practicing academic physicians.

Why would an educational institution or a renowned medical center want to acquire a medical school? At a superficial level a medical school guzzles money and certainly has the potential to bankrupt an educational institution. Why put the remainder the educational institution at risk? Many educational institutions of higher learning have achieved academic renown without having a medical school. Two such universities that immediately come to mind are Brandeis and Notre Dame. Indeed, in New York City universities such as Fordham and St. John's do not have medical schools. Even large, well-funded, universities keep their medical schools at arm's length financially. Medical schools constitute a unique academic breed, mixing a wide-ranging basic academic endeavor with direct service to people in need. Therefore, it is best for medical schools to be administered independently of the remaining educational entities that constitute the University. This is much more difficult for a small conglomerate of schools wherein the problems of the medical school make their way to the University's president on an almost daily basis.

Yet aside from financial considerations there were more cogent reasons for acquiring a medical school. First is the consideration that medicine is a noble profession dedicated to helping all human beings. If one posits that education is an endeavor that helps humanity then medical education may represent the highest form of this endeavor.

I wondered about the future of medical education and the pathways of creating a campus filled with intellectual ferment. The amount of knowledge bearing on human health that is being discovered by biomedical scientists all over the world on a daily basis is enormous and dwarfs the pace of advancement of medical knowledge that occurred previously in human history. It is too much to ask that medical students memorize the myriad metabolic cellular signal pathways that have been discovered in the last decade and, certainly, no one will have the particulars of the entire human genome that measures some 3 billion nucleotides, the building blocks of the genetic code, at their fingertips. Indeed, medicine has joined the other sciences in its reliance on computers as the repositories of its scientific data. Moreover, it is crucial to maintain the human approach of the physician to the patient based on the acquisition of a medical history and a hands-on physical examination. In time, it is not too outlandish to imagine, that the patient will be able to talk to a machine that will be programmed to ask sets of questions, record and digitize the reply, and present the physician with a completed history and a set of instructions for further diagnostic investigation. I believe that this would de-humanize medicine and prevent the establishment of a proper doctor-patient relationship so important for the care of the patient, but it is likely to happen.

Chapter 3. Musings on Medical Education

The fundamental educational question becomes how to manage the ever advancing knowledge base, and present the essences to the medical students, so that the students can stay abreast with the advance of the knowledge base throughout their professional lifetime. Perhaps one begins by laying down new assumptions about the role of physicians in the care of the patient. Medical care has moved from the first half of this century where the physician was the caregiver to a new era where the physician is part of a health care team that provides care to the patient. One prerogative of the physician already is being shared. Currently both physician assistants and nurse practitioners can write prescriptions. In hospitals the health care delivery team includes physicians, nurses, physician assistants, pharmacists and social workers. Even in the offices of private practitioners, physician assistants have assumed many of the roles of the physician in the care of the patient.

Now a new player must be added to the healthcare team and that is the computer in all its embodiments. First, patients' records on paper are being replaced by electronic records both in hospitals and in physicians' private offices. Secondly, it is too much to ask of the healthcare team to memorize all the details of a patient's care, including history, findings on physical examination, and laboratory test results. The ability to access all the patient's data at the patient's bedside without introducing errors of memory can only serve to improve patient care. It is reasonable to envisage that all healthcare workers will carry computer type instruments the size of a digital phone that contains all the up-to-date data concerning their patients. Moreover, consultation with an encyclopedic medical database is at the fingertips of the healthcare worker whether it be the dose of medication for a specific patient or the interactions of new medications needed for the patient and how to adjust for these interactions. When I was an intern in medicine at the Massachusetts General Hospital, the chairman of the department of medicine, the late Dr. Walter Bauer, when making rounds in the morning, would have the chief resident wheel several medical tomes in a cart so that the books could be consulted on specific questions and erroneous information not disseminated during medical rounds. This lesson, learned in my youth, has never been forgotten and I therefore welcome the advent of medical databases to be carried in every healthcare givers small computer. In the seminal discourse authored by René Descartes[1], the French philosopher, the imperfections of knowledge based on human memory are pointed out.

It is thus evident that medical students must be taught essentials that allow them to appreciate and consult with the present universe of medical knowledge. In this new era of personalized medicine, that is, healthcare given based on the specific genetic constitution of the individual patient, the singularity of each patient must be emphasized for the medical student. It is an ancient rabbinic dictum that the Almighty creates every soul with different attributes but all are equal before the Lord. In ensuing decades physicians will be adjusting medications according to the patient's individual genetic makeup and metabolic capabilities. The patient's gene sequences will be accessed from the physician's computer and the computer, at the touch of the physician's fingers, will supply the physician with lists of medications that would be applicable to this patient's genetic constitution.

There seems to be a logical approach to the sequence of educating a medical student. It begins with an understanding of the chemistry and functions of RNA and DNA, the biologic polymers that constitute the basic complex of the genetic code, RNA acting mainly as a first modifier and effector of the activity of the code. The second important code controllers are the proteins that provide a structural base for the huge DNA polymer and supply the enzymatic activities that control the expression of the code. Proteins, of course, also constitute the most important biologic material building blocks of living organisms. All of this must be presented in a manner that affords the medical student an in depth understanding of the interactions of structure and function. This perhaps is analogous to studying basic physical laws of mass and motion that can be applied to understanding the physics of new galaxies as they are discovered.

Redundancy and multiple controls of metabolic pathways are important components in maintaining the functionality of an organism. It is important for the medical student to be introduced to ontogeny early on so that the study of ontogeny goes hand-in-hand with the study of anatomical development and function based on the cellular structures that are fundamental to anatomical development. As organisms grow system networks are needed for communication and control, two of the major systems being the nervous system and the immune system. Signaling and signal control such as those mediated by hormones, and cytokines and chemokines the effector molecules of the immune system should be introduced as specific anatomic developments are discussed. The interaction of the organism with the environment must be taught at many levels, at the cellular level, at the specific organ level, at the total organism level and at the societal level. Organisms that are based on a DNA code share many fundamental characteristics but specifics vary. There do appear to be fundamental laws of biologic life that govern the development of all organisms indigenous to the planet Earth. Infectious diseases are assaults by other living organisms employing either a RNA or DNA code to usurp some of the cellular functions of the human host or to use the substances of the human host to multiply, spread and ensure the long-term viability of the invading organism.

Diseases should be introduced first at the level of genetic abnormalities resulting in heritable developmental diseases such as Tay-Sachs and Gaucher's diseases. The interaction of the environment, and the behavior of the human organism in relation to the environment, can then be introduced as an important component of the development of diseases during the lifetime of the individual.

Cellular senescence should be discussed as a fundamental issue of aging of the entire organism. Although, at present the root determination of longevity of the human organism is not understood, certain manifestations of the inexorable senescence of the organism, such as the progressive shortening of DNA repeats of the ends of the chromosomes, called telomeres, have been established. Senescence also has been tied to the activity of protein enzymes called sirtuins. These enzymes clip acyl molecules from the histones that are the proteins that surround the DNA in the nucleus and are important in the folding and control of function of the cellular DNA. Thus it is evident that an inexorable loss of DNA coding function is an important element of aging.

There are two interlocking compartments that comprise the development of a competent physician. First, there is the database of biomedical knowledge which is fundamental to the proper care of a patient. Second there is the human interaction of a physician with a patient. Although the computer now plays a central role in patient care it is critical to maintain that element of human interaction and human cogitation that no machine can ever replace. A physician must know how to interact and communicate with a patient. The two basic skills of history taking and physical examination must be inculcated into every physician. These are the foundations of the care provided by physicians to patients. It is these examinations, as part of the personal interaction of the physician with the patient, that allows the physician to individualize the medical care for that patient. In our present era of computer-based communication it is possible to send photographs of x-ray film, MRIs, CT scans, laboratory results, photographs and movies of patients. However, one cannot send the patient via phone lines, coaxial cables, or internet lines. There is always something missing in not being able to meet with the patient face-to-face and lay hands on the patient. The human nuances that are picked up by a savvy physician are important in establishing a gestalt of the patient. The computer can help the physician with the database for the patient, the database of medical knowledge that can be accessed through the computer, and in ease of processing paperwork for that patient. But the computer cannot substitute for that human element that probes and guides a patient through medical problems.

Chapter 4. Government and the Financing of Healthcare

The financing, and often the provision, of healthcare for the citizens of a governmental entity have become a societal responsibility. In Western Europe, especially, universal healthcare was an outgrowth of a movement towards Socialism following World War II. In the more socialistic countries the private practitioner of medicine is just about passé and the hospital and its clinics have become the providers of healthcare. At present, there are no compelling data to show any overall inferiority of social medicine compared to the private practice model of the United States in terms of patient well-being and longevity. It is probably more inconvenient to wait in a clinic waiting room or hospital emergency room in order to see the physician than to wait in a well-appointed private office where more courtesy is extended to the patient.

The Patient Protection and Affordable Care Act (ACA)[5] is a comprehensive health-care legislation that changes the entire landscape for healthcare delivery and services in the United States. This vast overhaul of health care begs for supporting scientific and operational data that unfortunately are lacking at present.

The first decade, certainly, of this new healthcare mandate will be an intensive learning experience, wherein the lesson plans will be created and multiply revised as the vicissitudes of the legislation's mandates are experienced and endured.

As one reads the many sections of the ACA, it becomes evident that the drafters of the legislation were aware that in so many instances they were entering uncharted waters. Therefore, the writers of the legislation created checkpoints at every turn to monitor the healthcare effectiveness, and cost-effectiveness, of each of the articles of the legislation. These checkpoints require actions by the federal, state and local governments, insurers, hospitals and private healthcare providers such as physicians in private practice.

The estimated cost of healthcare reform under the Affordable Care Act over the next 10 years is $940 billion. Much money will be expended by insurance companies, pharmaceutical firms, hospitals, healthcare practitioners, and state and local governments to develop the infrastructures and procedures to comply with the tenets of the new law, while maximizing the financial returns but minimizing the financial outlays. It is almost axiomatic to state that the insurance companies, the state and local governments, hospitals, healthcare practitioners, and the healthcare industry will turn, not to universities and academic medical institutions, but rather to qualified commercial entities to advise, guide and do much of the quality control, monitoring activities, research, and paperwork that is required by the new healthcare act.

The Affordable Care Act was drafted with full realization of the ignorance underlying much of the Act's approaches to delivery of health care. Thus one of the initial mandates of the ACA is the support of comparative effectiveness research by establishing a nonprofit Patient Centered Outcomes Research Institute. This mandate goes hand-in-hand with the requirement that all healthcare participants and providers monitor the effectiveness of their services.

Another first step mandate of the ACA is to create taskforces on Preventive Services and Community Preventive Services to develop, update and disseminate evidence-based recommendations on the use of clinical and community prevention services. It is important to be aware that consensus guidelines for delivery of proper preventive care to patients have not yet been formulated. It may take decades of trial and error approaches under the cloak of the ACA to develop effective standards of practice for preventive healthcare.

On January 1, 2014 the establishment of health insurance exchanges and subsidization of insurance premiums for individuals up to 400% of the poverty line, as well as single adults, took effect. Subsidies will be provided as advanceable, refundable tax credits. The states are required to monitor these insurance exchanges to determine both medical and cost-effectiveness in providing healthcare.

Another requirement in Section 3003 of the ACA is to create new types of reports and data analysis under the physician feedback program.

Stripped away of all the clauses and rhetoric, basic assumptions underlying the Affordable Care Act include:

1. We have to determine the best ways to deliver healthcare to the populace of the United States.
2. We must monitor the effectiveness of healthcare delivery and refine the methodology as the data are gathered and analyzed.
3. The quality of healthcare delivery must be monitored at all levels, and steps taken to ensure that quality care is maintained.
4. Healthcare providers will need to perform frequent self-assessments of effectiveness, quality and cost-effectiveness of healthcare delivery. In addition, these providers will be assessed periodically by outside agencies.
5. Healthcare providers will be rated as to performance.
6. The ratings will carry a financial impact.
7. Funds will be available for data acquisition and analysis needed to turn the ACA into an effective legislation.
8. The ACA sets the stage for:
    a) Dictating use of preferred drugs.
    b) Setting price controls, first on drugs and then on medical devices.
    c) Setting hospital and practitioner remunerations.
    d) Dictating standards of all healthcare practice.

Thus the Affordable Care Act4 that became law in 2010, to a large extent, represents an overhaul of medical care in the United States. One important element of this new congressional act is to make sure that there are sufficient numbers of healthcare workers to service the medical needs of the citizens of the United States. It is recognized that there do not exist sufficient numbers of physicians in the United States to care for all the people that would be eligible for medical care under the Act. The Act provides for the training of more primary care physicians. However, currently there appear to be insufficient numbers of allopathic medical schools (M.D. degree) and schools of osteopathic medicine (D.O. degree) to train the number of physicians that will be required to care for the citizens of the United States. Creating an academic allopathic medical school is a costly undertaking. A minimum of $250 million is needed to establish a credible academic allopathic medical school with proper research facilities and faculty.

There will be a push to create new facilities for the training of physicians in the United States. Signs of this push already are visible. Two commercial entities have applied to the Liaison Committee on Medical Education (LCME) of the American Medical Association for the approval of two for-profit allopathic medical schools. For the first time, the LCME has accepted the applications and will review the proposed medical schools. From what I can see, this represents an importation of the " teaching only" medical school model established by the for-profit medical school in Guadalajara, Mexico and the Ross and American Universities medical schools in the Caribbean. In essence, these offshore "medical degree mills" are not that different from most of the schools of osteopathic medicine that have been established in the United States. Well-run schools of osteopathic medicine are profitable and most bring some $6-$10 million annually to the bottom line. Protagonists of for-profit medical schools cite the large number of foreign trained medical students that serve as interns and residents in United States hospitals wherein most are graduates of medical schools in third world countries such as Bangladesh and Pakistan. These protagonists claim that the medical education provided by for-profit medical schools, and certainly by the existing schools of osteopathic medicine in the United States, is probably superior to that provided in many of the medical schools in third world countries.

If the LCME does approve the for-profit medical schools, I can foresee consequences that will effect major changes in medical education, and the perception of the physician, in the United States. In time, schools of osteopathic medicine will become allopathic schools. Osteopathic practice will undergo accepted clinical trials and those practices that are shown to have benefit for patients will be incorporated into the mainstream of medicine. There will be many more applications for for-profit medical schools. There will be two tiers of medical education in the United States. Physicians trained in "teaching only" schools will be looked upon as having a M.D. certificate rather than an M.D. academic degree. Many of the students attending academic medical schools will opt to enter joint M.D.-PhD programs in order to emphasize the quality and academic nature of their M.D. degree.

There is a major ramification of the need for more physicians that already is changing the way medical care is dispensed to the patient. Where formerly the physician was the major healthcare giver, healthcare now is provided increasingly by a team. The team approach was initiated in hospitals and has now entered the clinic and the physician's private office. In-hospital, the healthcare provider team may consist of the intern and resident physicians, the attending physician, the physician assistant or nurse practitioner, the registered nurse, the hospital pharmacist, the social worker, and the nurse's aide. On hospital wards the physician assistant or nurse practitioner has assumed many of the duties of the intern and resident physicians.

The question may be asked as to what difference there is in the type of care delivered by a physician assistant or nurse practitioner and an intern trained in a for-profit allopathic medical school or a school of osteopathic medicine. Let us consider some history. Several decades ago the question was raised in the UK whether medical students needed to be exposed to all that basic science in the medical school curriculum in order to become confident competent physicians. Indeed, why not emphasize clinical diagnostics and therapeutics from the very beginning so that the graduating medical students would be more competent in these areas. It was not clear that the in depth courses in the basic sciences had any effect on the ultimate competency of the physicians. This issue was never really resolved. Moreover, it is likely that as the physician assistants and nurse practitioners gather experience in practice they become more adept in the day-to-day care of patients both in hospital and in the private office. For-profit medical schools will argue that the greater coursework in the for-profit schools, compared to the curricula of schools for physician assistants and nurse practitioners, better prepares the student for a lifelong study of medicine.

The increasing governmental regulation of payments to physicians under the Affordable Care Act will force physicians to see more patients in order to maintain their incomes. This lack of time per patient will result in most of the hands on care of the patient being delivered by other members of the team such as the physician assistants, nurse practitioners and registered nurses. The dialogue between physician and patient, so important for proper patient care, will perforce decrease. It may well be that primary care will be delivered largely by physician assistants and nurse practitioners while physicians become even more specialized, providing specialized diagnoses and treatments such as surgery.

The Affordable Care Act emphasizes the need to provide "preventive care" for the citizens of the United States. The authors of the Act seemed to appreciate that at present there is no consensus definition of preventive care. It is reasonable to assume that preventive care would be cost-effective and should result in lower medical costs per citizen. The Act provides for the creation of a National Prevention Health Promotion and Public Health Council with an advisory group on prevention, health promotion and integrative public health. Funds will be provided for these new entities. These bodies will need to create the definitions of proper preventive care for the populace and construct the methodologies for testing the efficacy of their proposals for preventive care.

One fundamental aspect of preventive care is proper nutrition. The teaching of nutrition to health care workers, especially to medical students, must be revamped. The biology and chemistry of food substances needs to be emphasized in depth during the medical school training, especially during the first two years of the medical school curriculum. Indeed, teaching plant biology will help the medical student appreciate pharmacology and drug therapy in a more fundamental manner. Consumers are continuously bombarded with advertisements for "healthy foods" and with catalogs extolling the virtues of foods, herbs and "natural vitamins" derived from plants or animals. The physician needs to be fully acquainted with this area of human alimentation in order to properly guide the patient. Most food packaging includes rudimentary analysis of the chemical content and caloric load. The FDA may require even more detailed analysis of the foods. The physician needs to have the knowledge to guide the patient through this morass of health foods and food fads.

Quality monitoring is another important mandate of the Affordable Care Act. Hospitals, clinics and physicians private practices are directed to develop parameters for quality monitoring of their delivery of healthcare. Obviously, the development of universal standards for quality monitoring will require proper outcomes research undertakings in order to make data-based recommendations. At a fundamental level, every physician should practice self-questioning of whether the best care was delivered to the patient. Such continuous self-questioning will help prevent the physician from egregious errors in medical care and also will instill a sense of humility that is a necessary quality of a caring physician. Unfortunately, the human aspects of the physician patient relationship, and their therapeutic significance, probably will not be a part of the quality measures ultimately mandated by the Affordable Care Act.

23

Chapter 5. Financial Pressures in the System

One of the major objectives of the Affordable Care Act is to rein in rising health care costs. Initiatives already launched by states such as Massachusetts, that created legislation to extend medical care to all state citizens, address the fundamental problem of cost containment. The Affordable Care Act establishes Accountable Care Organizations (ACOs) that are responsible for monitoring and overseeing the dispensing of medical care in their networks. Traditionally in the United States outpatient medical care was given by private practitioners who in essence are in the business of running a privately owned medical practice. The advantage of such a system is that the physician who is the owner of the practice must attract and maintain the loyalty of the patient, as the consumer and the means of revenue, for the business. This is the basis of the personal care that characterized medical practice in this country. Under governmental pressures for cost containment the business of medicine slowly will change its character in the United States. The common method of payment to physicians until now has been the fee for service model. Obviously, the more services rendered by a physician to the patient the more fees will be garnered by the physician. A new model that is slowly infiltrating medical payment is the global payment model. In this model the State or insurance company will give the physician a flat fee to care for the patient. If the costs for caring for the patient are less than budgeted for the patient the physician will be rewarded with a bonus or incentive payment. Under this method of payment there is an incentive for the physician to control costs in order to obtain the financial reward. Ultimately, the physician's income will be determined by a governmental body. The solo practitioner is likely to disappear. Physicians are combining into very large groups in order to have more clout in their negotiations with insurance companies and governmental bodies. In addition, more and more physicians are joining group practices under the aegis of hospital groups or medical schools. The final financial rewards to the physician may be lower but the physician will not need to deal with all the paperwork, billing problems and governmental regulations that will be centrally handled by the hospital or medical school. At present, there appears to be no compelling evidence that fee for service payment results in any better medical outcomes than a global payment method.

In order to expand the medical coverage of the populace in the United States and to control medical costs, the Affordable Care Act emphasizes and promotes the training of primary care physicians. It is expected that the cost of a visit to a primary care physician will be less expensive and that such physicians will assume a much larger patient load in order to achieve a respectable income. Payments to primary physicians will be monitored and periodically adjusted to provide respectable incomes. Gradually medical practice in the United States will more and more resemble European type medical practice in which the medical specialist is part of a hospital group rather than a private practice. Fewer medical specialists, whose incomes now are set by the hospital or medical school, should lower the overall costs of medical practice in the United States. Governmental control over healthcare further is increased by the monitoring of the number of healthcare workers and students, including doctors and nurses, by a National Healthcare Workforce Commission and a National Center for Healthcare Workforce Analysis. Another objective of the Affordable Care Act is to help students from disadvantaged groups enter the healthcare industry thus promoting diversity amongst healthcare workers.

Individual states will shape primary care for their citizens. For example, in December of 2011 Washington State's Healthcare Authority announced that it intended to stop paying for emergency department visits by Medicaid beneficiaries when those visits were deemed unnecessary for an emergency department and should have been handled by a primary care office. Yet the Federal Emergency Medical Treatment and Active Labor Act[6] requires emergency rooms to see and stabilize all patients in need.

If the government can keep the population healthy, then the need for costly health care decreases. Therefore, another important objective of the Affordable Care Act is to encourage the study of public health with the ultimate goal of applying what is learned to the overall improvement of the health of the citizens of the United States. Public health science tracks are supported with emphasis on advanced degrees in public health, epidemiology and emergency preparedness response. In time, public health considerations will pervade just about every aspect of a person's life in the United States.

What should an individual expect from the changes in healthcare that are being legislated through the Affordable Care Act and separately by individual states? First, let us compare the health of citizens of the United States with that of Western Europe where health care is given through socialized medicine. In terms of final outcomes, the life spans of citizens in the United States are not longer than that of citizens of Western European countries with socialized medicine. Although it may be argued that the overall average numbers in the United States are decreased by poor numbers from a significant portion of the populace that at present is not covered by the health care system, it also can be argued that such population mixes exist in every country. Acquisition of medical care, especially non-urgent medical care, is less convenient for the patient in countries with socialized medicine but emergency needs seem to be well handled by the hospitals. Moreover, the medical schools in Europe appear to have sufficient student applications although the incomes of physicians in Europe may be smaller than that of physicians in the United States. It seems that ultimately the models for providing health care are determined by what the country can afford financially.

A careful perusal of the Affordable Care Act leaves one with the impression that the authors of this legislation were well aware that the outcomes and effectiveness of the health care models proposed under the legislation were to a large extent unknown and unproved. At almost every step in the implementation of this legislation the authors built-in support for the outcomes research that would be necessary in order to establish the validity of the health care models. The logical conclusion is that there will be many missteps along the way and that it will be many years before a really effective healthcare model will be pervasive in the United States.

Do advances in medical science and medical practice contribute to increasing healthcare costs? This is a very important question. For example, with the development of the technology for determining the genetic composition of organisms, including humans, there has been an emphasis on the practice of what is called personalized medicine. A common example is the determination of the type of kinase called K-ras, that is a phosphorylase enzyme, present in a colonic tumor in order to choose the proper chemotherapeutic agent to treat that tumor. Such determinations are at present expensive. It may be envisioned, that sometime in the future every person will have a determination of their genetic profile so that throughout their lifetime their medical treatment will be personalized. The cost of the one-time determination of the genetic profile will be offset by the savings accrued throughout the person's life because proper medications dictated by their particular genetic makeup will be chosen when they need medical therapy.

How does one approach the cost-effective education of medical students in the current four year duration of schooling as the volume of medical knowledge continues to increase almost exponentially. The present teaching approach to medical students is based upon the 1910 Flexner report. The rapid advance in medical science and its translation into treatments for patients since 1910 and especially since the end of World War II mandates that methodology and curricula of medical education are overhauled. Attendance at daily lectures becomes redundant when those lectures can be available on one's computer and all assignments, the research necessary to find the data for completion of those assignments, also can be effected through the use of computers. Indeed, many European physicians obtained degrees and built important careers in medicine and medical science with hardly any attendance at lectures during their medical school years relying on textbooks and lecture notes provided by the medical school faculty. Lecture attendance was not mandatory in many European medical schools but students were required to pass exams. There are those who argue that in order to make even basic science lessons relevant for medical students that those lessons could be built around a clinical presentation. I am not convinced that such an approach is necessary for what now constitutes a core understanding of biochemistry and molecular biology. I believe that it is necessary for medical students to be aware of and understand basic biologic mechanisms with the underlying chemistry, physics and molecular biology. On the other hand, I do believe that it is important to introduce medical students to real patients during the first year of schooling. This hands-on experience can be supplemented by watching patient interviews, history taking, physical examinations and some laboratory examinations on computers.

Chapter 6. Quality Healthcare Delivery

Given the emphasis of the Affordable Care Act on measuring effectiveness and quality of health care it becomes important to inculcate rules of behavior that favor delivery of quality care from the very beginning of the medical school education. Education should build character. Self-assessment must be built into every act undertaken by a physician and the medical student must be taught to include an assessment of quality in every note written on a patient. The medical student must come to feel that the student's prime responsibility in life, a life that the student voluntarily has chosen, is to ensure the welfare of the patient.

The student must be taught to appreciate the physician's responsibility both to the quantity and quality of life of the patient. In helping patients to make so-called end-of-life decisions the physician must be able to balance the two elements, the quantity versus the quality, of life. Of utmost importance, every physician must feel that every moment of a person's life is precious and that the physician must battle to preserve every moment of the patient's life. With this in mind, the physician will be better able to aid patients and their families in their quests to care for their family members in their aged and physically declining years. I believe that it is the duty of society to care for the aged, as it is to care for the helpless and disabled, and to provide the mental and physical needs that should dignify the waning years of a human's existence. In helping patients and their families to make critical health care decisions the physician must learn how to empathize, commiserate, and even feel the pain that may be wracking the patient. Of course, some medical students are emotionally better able to deal with patients but the continued teaching of these human skills should be basic to the medical school education. In a sense the physician becomes part of one's family and a very important family member at that.

How does the physician deal with the patient, as an experimental subject, in a clinical trial? The underlying ethics of a clinical trial is the volunteerism of the patient subject. Fundamentally, the patient is offering themselves for the ultimate help of others and, hopefully, also of themselves. Yet during the conduct of a randomized, controlled, blinded trial the patient may be receiving no more than a placebo whose only therapeutic effect may be the so-called placebo effect in mitigating the patient's symptoms. The medical student must be made to understand that as the student is offering their life for the welfare of others the patient who agrees to enter a clinical trial is making a similar offering. Society advances when people help each other. Therefore, I take exception to those who posit that blinded clinical trials are unethical because some patients will be receiving only placebo. It would be unethical to give patients medications and treatments whose effectiveness and safety were not established by proper clinical trials.

In his work, a Discourse on the Method of Rightly Conducting the Reason and Seeking the Truth in the Sciences[1], the famed French philosopher Rene Descartes stated that words were inexact and that the precision of numbers led to the conclusion that mathematics was the language of God. Indeed, mathematics is the basis of all of the exact sciences. Although the practice of medicine has been termed both an art and a science numbers are increasingly becoming the basic language of medicine. The ability to measure relative risks is fundamental to the proper practice of medicine. For example, when prescribing a medication for an illness such as heart failure the physician will consider the numbers that characterize the risk of not treating the patient, compared to the risk of an untoward effect from the medication. The benefit of treatment, often expressed as the percentage of patients with a given type and stage of illness that will respond to treatment positively, must significantly outweigh the risks posed by the potential side effects of the treatments used, also often expressed as the percentage of patients who developed the different side effects associated with a medication. Perhaps the art of medicine is the skill in weighing the numbers and making the best therapeutic decisions for the patient. There are no real absolutes in medicine. Indeed, humans do not deal with absolutes. The core of even the exact sciences such as physics is dealing with numbers that represent probability values.

The Affordable Care Act turns the gauging of effectiveness of healthcare deliveries into expressions of relative numbers, usually recorded as percentages. Thus a given approach to extending insurance to uninsured citizens may reach only 70% of the intended population. These numbers will be tracked by entities established under the Affordable Care Act. Physicians will express the monitoring of the quality of the health care they give to their patients in number form. In summary, when all the elements of the Affordable Care Act are in place the effectiveness of healthcare delivery in the United States will be expressed in number form both for the overall effort and for the specific parts.

Chapter 7. Healthcare at the Poles of Life

The two poles of life, childhood and aging, pose the most daunting hurdles for the delivery of healthcare. The first stage of life begins with the developing fetus and it will be important for pregnant women to receive proper prenatal care. An effort must be made to significantly decrease perinatal mortality in the United States. Children are dependent on their parents for ensuring that they are receiving proper care. All parents must be induced to bring their children to healthcare facilities for proper vaccination and preventive care, including dental care. The schooling of a child should not be hampered because the parents do not recognize that the child requires glasses to adjust vision. The diets of children are determined by parents and the prevention of childhood obesity begins with the parents. Children are often the subject of accidental trauma that may be caused by parents' neglect of childhood safety measures in the home and at play.

Caring for persons at the other pole of life, the aged, poses even more complex and financially costly problems. The communication problems posed by many aged patients are more difficult than those posed by a toddler not yet speaking. The abilities of the aged patient are waning while the abilities of the toddler are growing. It is axiomatic that it is less expensive to care for a patient in the patient's home. It usually is also more dignified for the patient.

The question of who will care for the increasing number of elderly citizens of the United States is to a large extent dependent on the question of what the healthcare team will look like in future decades. If the Affordable Care Act does add 30 million people to the insured pool, the present health care system will be overtaxed and ill-prepared to extend the mandated care to this new group of patients. First, there are insufficient numbers of physicians in the United States to care for another 30 million people. Secondly, new facilities will have to be built to provide the hospitals and clinics for the care of these added patients. This is costly and the government will make great effort to defray much of the cost from the existing healthcare system. I can envision the following scenario. It is costly to educate physicians, whether allopathic or osteopathic, and physicians expect to be remunerated at a relatively high pay scale. Therefore, the question can be asked whether physicians are really necessary to deliver the hands-on day-to-day care required to deal with the more common health problems that precipitate most visits to family physicians. It is likely that physician assistants, properly trained, at a lower cost, and expecting smaller payments for their professional services than physicians, can deliver the day-to-day mundane medical care including monitoring patients and running preventive care programs. The physician assistants can team with a nurse practitioner or a registered nurse to care for most of the daily needs of patients. I believe this would be a better solution than creating two classes of physician, those who practice in hospitals and those who practice in outpatient settings and do not have hospital admitting privileges. Under such a system physicians outside of the hospital system become more like trades-people rather than academic professionals. However, if there is a proliferation of for-profit medical schools in the United States then one can predict that there will be two classes of physicians, the more academic hospital physician and the more trades-like outpatient physician.

The first objective in the care of the elderly is to try to maintain the patient in the home environment. There are many visiting nurse services that provide in-home visits to patients. During these visits the nurse may inject the patient with medications, such as insulin for diabetic patients, and record the results of the superficial examination including the vital signs-blood pressure, pulse, respiratory rate and temperature. It would make sense to include a physician assistant or nurse practitioner as the key professional to visit the patient to oversee home healthcare. Physicians no longer want to make home visits and the costs of such visits would be too expensive. A physician assistant can do a more complete and more informed history and physical examination than a nurse and also prescribe medication. I believe that a physical therapist should be an important member of the home care team of the elderly patient and that elderly patients should undergo a physical therapy session for 45 minutes at least three times a week. Physical therapy sessions contribute to the patient's well-being and mobility. Caring for the elderly patient in a home setting is more dignified, is more cost-effective and is likely to provide better maintenance of the patient's health than would residence in a nursing home or chronic hospital setting.

Chapter 8. Informed Patients

Given the increasing complexity of medical care it is important for patients to have informed advocates to help the patient navigate the health system and make informed decisions. Most lay persons cannot deal with the technical medical data thrown at them by their physicians. A more informed advocate is required to explain matters to the patient and help the patient in decision-making for the patient's continued healthcare. The advocate may be a family member, a friend or a professional that is paid for such services. Patients face real difficulties in making decisions, both at the emotional level and at the level of information, when faced with the request to sign a do not resuscitate (DNR) order or to choose a proper health care proxy. A patient advocate can be very helpful in these situations. Moreover, the interaction of the patient advocate with physicians in an outpatient setting and with ward personnel in the hospital perforce will move the health care givers to pay more attention to that patient.

Are hospitals whose faculty members are engaged in research projects necessarily the best medical institutions in which a patient should seek clinical care? Certainly physicians in hospitals that treat large numbers of patients are more likely to be clinically facile in both diagnosis and treatment. The more academic institutions whose faculty members are engaged in research are more likely to be able to bring to bear the most current diagnostic modes and therapies, especially for diseases that are being studied at that particular institution. For example, patients with cancers who have failed standard therapies are more likely to be able to receive promising new drugs that are being investigated in clinical trials at research institutions. On the other hand, if the patient is to have a cardiac pacemaker placed the patient should seek out a hospital that places such devices daily. Experience is still the best teacher for hands-on medical diagnosis and therapy.

Chapter 9. Future Healthcare in the United States

What is likely to become of healthcare in the United States? The government slowly but inexorably will assume control of healthcare in a modified social medicine type model. Indeed, for several decades the government has been the underpinnings for the financing of healthcare in the United States. Whether one considers government financing of students beginning with loans for college and medical school tuitions, the support of hospitals, the provision of funds for Medicaid and Medicare, the support of residency training programs in hospitals and the support of public health programs, the control of healthcare by the government is pervasive. The recent establishment of a National Institutes of Health for Translational Research, emphasizing the development and clinical trials of new therapies, will allow the federal government ultimately to control of the costs of medications. When the government provides funds to investigate a new drug and facilitates clinical trials with that drug, the involvement of the government will translate into setting the costs to the consumer when the drug is marketed. This will provide the federal government with great leverage on the pharmaceutical companies and will afford the government an important hand in controlling the revenue and profits of the pharmaceutical industry. Such leverage on the pharmaceutical industry ultimately will help to control rising health care costs and serve to decrease costs for the care of the elderly who consume multiple medications daily.

The Affordable Care Act makes the healthcare environment even more unfavorable for the private practitioner of medicine. The Act mandates reports to the federal government, electronic record-keeping, monitoring of quality control and the filling out the many different forms that would financially overburden a solo practitioner. Therefore, physicians increasingly are forming large groups so that the government reporting costs can be shared and more leverage would be present in negotiations with insurance payers. Such group practices may have hundreds of physician members. Hospitals are buying up medical practices to ensure practice related income, leverage in negotiating with insurance companies for payments and to provide a steady flow of patients to occupy hospital beds and hospital services such as rehabilitation, cardiovascular diagnosis and treatment, and surgery. One of the ramifications of this change in medical practice will be that the physician of the patient will no longer be available all day and all week. Night time and weekend problems probably will require a trip to a hospital emergency room or to a hospital clinic set up to treat such visits. Physicians, whether in group practices or in hospital or faculty practices, will be given the opportunity to earn more money if they see more patients. The government will provide bonus payments to physicians based on the number of patients seen, the lowering of costs per patient of diagnostic and therapeutic interventions and by providing evidence of quality care based on the parameters set by the government.

Will the increasing control of the government on the financial life of the physician result in fewer student applications to medical schools? I do not believe that the effects on medical school enrollments will be material. First, medical school applications in countries where socialized medicine was instituted have not reduced significantly the numbers of students applying to medical schools. Secondly, economic expectations and anticipations of financial rewards are dampened as the system changes. There always will be need for more physicians as the population increases and the physician will be happy to be needed and to look forward to durable employment. Thirdly, the practice of medicine gives personal satisfactions to the practitioners with direct hands-on help for other human beings, that is not easily found in other professions. Therefore, there always will be dedicated physicians whose objective in life is to bring healing and solace to other human beings. Nevertheless, the practice of medicine increasingly will become a 9 to 5 job buttressed by physicians who will staff emergency rooms or specialized clinics in the night time hours.

There is a lurking danger to patients, and to the mores of society, as a result of total governmental control of healthcare. Will governmental rules dictate who receives healthcare and who does not, or at the very least who receives assiduous healthcare and who is largely neglected? Elderly patients, especially, may be subject to such decisions given the financial burdens of caring for the elderly. Such discussions already have arisen more than a decade ago amongst members of a congressional committee dealing with health care issues. The late Dr. Thomas Thomas Chalmers, who then was president and CEO of the Mount Sinai medical Center in New York City, was vehemently opposed to any such discussions. The basic role of the physician is to battle for every moment of life and not to decide who lives and who dies. It is crucial for any national health care plan to treat the elderly with dignity, concern and compassion.

What will the healthcare system look like in the United States 2 to 3 decades from now? Already in 1980, Dr. Arnold Relman, the former editor of the prestigious New England Journal of Medicine, warned about the rise of the new "medical industrial complex".[3] Dr. Relman was commenting on the great rise of a new industry that supplies health care services for profit including proprietary hospitals and nursing homes, diagnostic laboratories, home care and emergency room services, and hemodialysis. Such profit-based services tend to seek ever-increasing profits resulting in overuse and fragmentation of healthcare services. Dr. Relman warned that this rising industry would result in increasing healthcare costs. In a more recent article published in the British Medical Journal in 2012,[4] Dr. Relman warned that the healthcare system in the United States is headed for financial disaster. Rising medical costs have the potential to bankrupt the entire healthcare system in the United States. In a perspective overview of 200 years of hospital costs and mortality at the Massachusetts General Hospital published in the June 7, 2012 issue of the New England Journal of Medicine[2] the adjusted cost per patient alive at discharge began to rise steeply in the late 1950s. Of note, since 2001, although mortality has been level, the cost per patient has continued to increase greatly. Dr. Relman3 predicted these events and saw the root of the problem as the development of the healthcare system in the United States into a profit driven industry. Therefore, in order to bring financial stability to the healthcare system in the United States federal legislation would be necessary to wring out the profit motive from healthcare.[3,4] The Affordable Care Act does not address the core of the financial problem of healthcare. One of the basic corrective moves would be to turn physicians into salaried employees. The price of drugs would be regulated by the federal government and drug development would be partially financed by the federal government. The United States spends more on health care per capita than other developed countries. Yet some 50 million denizens of the United States do not have any medical coverage and many patients do not have access to the best healthcare. Indeed, healthcare in the United States may not be better than healthcare in countries that spend much less. In the US physicians are in business and medical care constitutes a large industry at $2.7 trillion or 18% of the US economy. The healthcare industry pays for marketing efforts to induce physicians and the patient consumer to use drugs, laboratory tests and all sorts of devices. All seek to maximize revenue and prices are not regulated. Fraudulent billing adds to the cost of healthcare representing some 5 to 10% of the costs. So-called defensive medicine is practiced by many physicians in order to avoid malpractice suits by patients; this results in overuse of diagnostic services adding to the overall costs of healthcare in the United States.

It is difficult to state with any certainty that if 50 million persons were added to the healthcare roles of U. S. population that this would result in an acute shortage of physicians. Some experts argue that there is no overall shortage of physicians in the United States but that there is a maldistribution of physicians that leaves many areas of the United States with poor medical coverage. As I previously stated, it would be more economical to use physicians' assistants and nurse practitioners as frontline healthcare deliverers.

It is inevitable that as the delivery of healthcare in the United States becomes more socialized that the nature and role of the primary care physician, whether family physician or internist, will change. It is likely that there will be two castes of physicians, namely, those that practice in hospital or in academic medical institutions and those that see patients only on an outpatient basis. This already is the portrait of physicians practicing in Western Europe and other countries, such as Israel, where there are two types of physicians those that see only outpatients and those that practice in hospitals and the medical school associated medical centers. The latter are considered the expert physicians while the former are there to take care of what would be considered routine, outpatient day-to-day patient needs. The role of even the internist in the United States is slowly changing. Physicians who recommend hospitalization for their patients increasingly are discovering that in hospital the patients are taken care of by hospitalists who have assumed the role previous played by internists who hospitalized their patients, and by specialists in the various specialty departments of the hospital. Thus the continuity of care, both as outpatient and in-patient, that was the hallmark of medical practice in the United States and was considered to be a key determinant of the excellence of medical care in the United States, is slowly disappearing. Thus from entry into the emergency room where the patient is evaluated by a physician certified in emergency medicine, to care on the wards of the hospital where the patient is taken care of by hospitalists certified in hospital medicine, the role of the primary care physician, whether certified in family medicine or internal medicine, is negligible.

In the future, how will patients choose physicians? Will the patient contact the local Accountable Care Organizations (ACO), established under the rules of the Affordable Care Act, to obtain a referral to a primary care physician or will the patient just appear in one of the large practices and ask to be seen by a physician? The local primary physician will slowly disappear and patients will access physicians in accord with the provisions of the Affordable Care Act. In many areas of the country physician groups have established walk-in clinics where patients can go for outpatient care as needed. In most countries where medicine is socialized outpatient care is delivered by large clinics funded and operated by governmental agencies. Since patients usually do not see the same physician at every outpatient visit the delivery of healthcare becomes less personal.

In order to significantly slow the relentless rise in healthcare costs it is imperative to discontinue the use of unapproved diagnostic modalities and therapies. Outcomes research will be required to examine the medical effectiveness, and the cost-effectiveness, of commonly prescribed diagnostic and therapeutic interventions. The need for outcomes research to examine the gamut of medical practice largely is built into the Affordable Care Act. Suggested, or rather prescribed, diagnostic and therapeutic approaches to ailments produced by government agencies, based on the results of outcomes research projects, will become the guidelines for physicians in treating patients. The pressure to reduce the financial burden by eliminating wasteful ineffective medical practices will move the government to control the application of medical practice to patients. Such outcomes research was recently at play in the revised suggestions for the discontinuation of the almost routine use of the measurement of the blood level of prostatic specific antigen (PSA) to screen for prostatic cancer. Instead of including the PSA test amongst the routine blood tests drawn on male patients older than 45 years of age the physician will consider carefully whether there is a need for a PSA determination in this specific patient. Currently it is projected that healthcare spending as a share of the gross domestic product (GDP) will reach 20.1% by 2021. The Agency for Healthcare Research and Quality will attempt to develop methods to decrease the current rise in healthcare costs. Local accountable care organizations set up under the Affordable Care Act will be the first-line in the battle to contain rising healthcare costs. It also has been suggested that the United States would be divided into geographic areas called Health Improvement Communities (HIC) essentially to bundle the accountable care organizations into larger supervising units attempting to provide cost-effective care to the populace of the United States. It is hoped that by ensuring that low care patient costs are actually low care costs, the resources will be available to care for those patients that are actually high cost care patients.

Let us consider the healthcare services infrastructure that will be necessary to deliver universal health care to the citizens of the United States. Let us begin with medical students and medical schools. Since the physician in future decades will likely be a salaried employee and the economic return from future practice that may justify a $40-$50,000 yearly tuition costs will be absent, tuition costs will have to be lowered or subsidized by the federal government in order to graduate sufficient physicians to deliver universal health care. Governmental support for the academics of medical schools, that is the research that determines the academic standing and reputation of a medical school, will increase very slowly, and the private sector will increasingly fund biomedical research. The medical student will need to be inculcated with the team approach to medical care and to the defined role of the physician as a team member. The physician may be the ultimate medical authority of the team but much of the necessary knowledge and data will be carried in a small handheld computer. Healthcare teams that include primary care physicians may be assigned geographic areas in which the team will visit patients in their home. This will be very important in future years for the care of the increasing number of elderly patients in the United States. The federal government will determine how many physicians, physician assistants and nurse practitioners, pharmacists, and physical therapists are graduated each year to serve the needs of the population of the United States. In order to save costs medical schools will rely on 33 online and computer aided instruction while decreasing the number of faculty. As smaller federal grant awards, fewer and smaller philanthropic donations and lower financial support from associated hospitals squeeze the finances of medical schools, the schools increasingly will seek to balance their budgets according to tuition revenues.

As the government endeavors to develop and finance a workable health care program the pharmaceutical industry will be facing a crisis. The pipeline of new drugs is becoming smaller. Patents on blockbuster drugs are expiring and the drugs are being marketed by generic drug companies. The government increasingly will control the pricing of new drugs. These factors will place a financial burden on the pharmaceutical companies and curtail the financial outlays that are required to develop new drugs. Pharmaceutical companies already are slimming down and are cutting the number of employees. In order to maintain a pipeline of new drugs the pharmaceutical industry will need to interact with academia and fund research in academic institutions, especially schools of medicine, to develop the basic science and animal pharmacokinetic and therapeutic effectiveness of new drug candidates. Large pharmaceutical firms increasingly will turn to new biotechnology companies to acquire drug pipelines. Therefore, as financial stresses on the national government impact financing of research grants the pharmaceutical industry will need to step in to finance the advances in basic biomedical science that are the foundations of the discovery of new drugs.

The Pharmaceutical industry will face other stresses. The Affordable Care Act mandates the collection of better predictive data for costs and outcomes. The Patient Protection and Affordable Care Act's rules on benefit design and minimum loss ratios will further crimp the insurance industry's tight margins. Insurers perforce will turn to the creation of models for future disease progression and response to therapy as they consider the design of products offered to clients. Pharmaceutical firms will need to provide data for their drugs that enable such predictions. The financing of healthcare increasingly will rely on value driven models. Pharmaceutical companies will need to assess comparative economics in their drug development business plans and consider how their drug products affect patient health outcomes and overall cost of care. The development and marketing of "me-too" drugs will no longer be worthwhile financially. Indeed, investigation of comparative effectiveness of drugs, based on outcomes data, will become standard in the pharmaceutical industry.

The rise and expansion of Accountable Care Organizations will limit the ability of pharmaceutical sales representatives to meet with physicians. Pharmaceutical firms will need to find new avenues of marketing to physicians and patients. Presentation of comparative data of drug effectiveness and toxicity, based on outcomes research, will be integrated into these new marketing presentations. The Affordable Care Act includes the establishment of an independent payment advisory board, and federally funded outcomes research to provide the data necessary to make informed decisions. Proper outcomes research in all facets of drug development will be crucial for pharmaceutical firms to drive sales of medications.

Non-communicable diseases that are often chronic afflictions plague the aging population. Diseases such as rheumatoid and osteoarthritis, stroke, angina pectoris, diabetes mellitus, chronic lung disease, asthma, hypertension and cataracts exert a great financial burden on society. There are various approaches that will be used in concert to address the burden of non-communicable diseases. This includes an integrated primary care approach to the care of the patient, programs for disease prevention and accountability organizations to monitor and ensure the application of proper care to the patients. For example, infections such as human papilloma virus, Helicobacter pylori, hepatitis B virus and hepatitis C virus account for some 16-18% of cancers. Smoking is associated both with cancer and heart disease. Unhealthy diets are associated with heart disease, hypertension and diabetes mellitus. Effective prevention programs could decrease the incidence and financial burdens of these diseases. Medical students will have to be imbued with the need for preventive care on a societal level and the application of preventive care to the individual patient.

Chapter 10. Healthcare in Crisis. Why Should a University Have a Medical School?

I have painted a picture of a healthcare system in crisis. There are two aspects to this crisis. First, there is the problem of delivering proper healthcare to all denizens of the United States and the even greater problem of financing the healthcare system. So now the question of why a university would want to purchase a medical school becomes even more trenchant.

This question led to very lively discussions between myself and my late dear friend Dr. Bernard Lander. Let us reframe the question. Why would a university emphasizing this study of the humanities want to purchase a medical school? The answer to this question is rather simple. The essential objective of medicine and the health sciences is to serve human beings. Therefore, should not the study of medicine fit into the rubric of the study of the humanities? The statement that the practice of medicine is both an art and a science has been repeated so many times that it now has become a cliché. I believe that it is more correct to say that the practice of medicine is an art based on science. Let us consider the essential roles of education in general. Obviously, human beings are educated in schools in order to gain knowledge that will allow them to function in society and to contribute to the economic well-being of society. Yet there may be a more fundamental role for education and that is to build character. Kindness and service to other human beings should be cultivated into every student as the student is introduced to history, the arts and the sciences. The acquisition and expansion of knowledge should be viewed as the road to create better human beings. The underlying reason for pursuing a career in medicine should always be the realization that the most noble activity of a human being is to dedicate one's life to serving and helping others. Therefore, it is understandable that Dr. Bernard Lander, a social scientist, who also was a clergyman, should believe that it was his mission to establish a medical school as part of his endeavors in education.

In attempt to create more caring and dedicated physicians during the years of medical education should courses in the humanities be taught, and required, to medical students? The study of the history of medicine itself is replete with heartwarming examples of physicians who sacrificed their lives for the benefit of humanity. I believe that courses in the history of medicine should be mandatory as part of the medical school curriculum. It is important for medical students not only to understand medical knowledge and practice but also to be able to meld their own dedication to their patients with the history of past physicians. My dear friend and I shared the vision of creating both very knowledgeable and very caring physicians.

Bibliography

1. Descartes, Rene. Discourse on the Method of Rightly Conducting the Reason and Seeking the Truth in the Sciences. Maryland: Wildside Press, 2008.

2. Meyer, Gregg S., Denehin, Akinluw A., Liu, Xiu, Neuhauser, Duncan. "Two Hundred Years of Hospital Costs and Mortality-MGH and Four Eras of Value in Medicine," New England Journal of Medicine 366, no. 23 (2012), 2147-49.

3. Relman, Arnold. "The Medical- Industrial Complex," New England Journal of Medicine 303, no. 17 (1980), 963-70.

4. Relman, Arnold, " Why the US Healthcare System Is Failing and What Might Rescue It," British Medical Journal 344 (2012), e3052.

5. US Congress. The Patient Protection and Affordable Care Act. Public Law 111-148 (2010), H. R. 3590.

6. 42 US Congress. Emergency Medical Treatment and Labor Act. (1986), 1395dd.

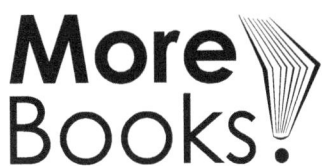
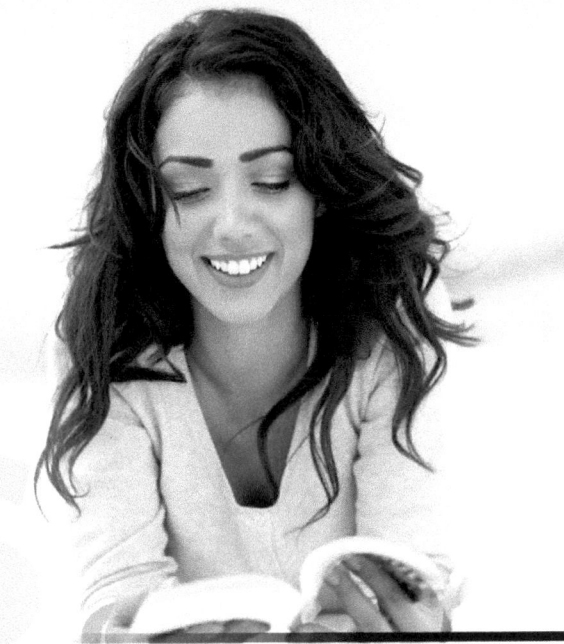

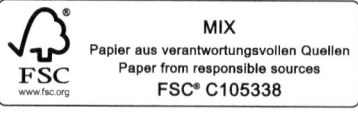

Printed by Books on Demand GmbH, Norderstedt / Germany